T0231087

QUALITY RULES
in
STERILE PRODUCTS MANUFACTURE

REVISED
AMERICAN EDITION

John Sharp

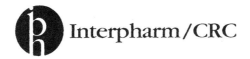 Interpharm/CRC

Boca Raton   London   New York   Washington, D.C.

Visit the CRC Press Web site at www.crcpress.com

© 2002 by John Sharp
Interpharm is an imprint of CRC Press

No claim to original U.S. Government works
International Standard Book Number 1-57491-134-1
Printed in the United States of America 1 2 3 4 5 6 7 8 9 0
Printed on acid-free paper

CONTENTS

Preliminary Note for Training Managers and Instructors

My earlier booklet entitled *Quality Rules—A Short Guide to GMP* was published in response to an evident need for a simple, readable account of the essentials of current Good Manufacturing Practice. That the need was a real one has been confirmed by the high and continuing demand for copies. Recently, a revised, special American Edition of that first booklet in the "Quality Rules" series has been published by Interpharm Press. That was followed by the American Edition of *Quality Rules in Packaging*. This present text is thus the third booklet in the series of "Quality Rules," American Editions.

Although brief early mention is made of the basic ideas of Quality and GMP, it is assumed that the reader is aware of the fundamentals of these concepts, as set out in *Quality Rules—A Short Guide to Drug Products GMP*. It is important that trainees are aware that the special GMP requirements for sterile products manufacture are *additional* to, not separate from, or alternative to "general" GMP requirements. These apply to *all* healthcare products—drug products, medical devices, diagnostics, APIs, and so on. When these products have to be sterile, then there are additional requirements. These additional requirements are what this present booklet is about. There are two reasons why it is called "Quality Rules. . . ." It *does* contain some rules about Quality. But it also means that "Quality Rules," in the sense that Quality is tops, or the best, just as some people might say "The White Sox Rule," or "Broncos Rule," and so on.

As with all the booklets in this series, this one is intended to be used in conjunction with appropriate training programs, and to provide the trainee with a basic outline to keep as a reminder, a refresher, and a reference.

John Sharp
December 2001

1. QUALITY AND STERILE PRODUCTS

This booklet is about making products that have to be STERILE. Specifically, it is about GOOD MANUFACTURING PRACTICE (GMP) in the manufacture of products that have to be sterile, products like:

- INJECTIONS, for example:
    - Some antibiotics,
    - Large volume infusions ("drips"),
  and
    - Vaccines.
(Another name for Injections is "Parenterals.")

- EYE PRODUCTS, for example:
    - Eye drops,
    - Eye lotions,
  and
    - Eye ointments.
(Another name for Eye Products is "Ophthalmic Products" or just "Ophthalmics.")

- EAR DROPS.

- SOME SKIN PREPARATIONS, for example:
    - Lotions, creams, and ointments for application to broken skin.

- IRRIGATION SOLUTIONS, for example:
    - Wound irrigations
and
    - Bladder irrigations.

- IMPLANTS.

- MANY DRESSINGS.

- MEDICAL and SURGICAL DEVICES and INSTRUMENTS.

- MANY DIAGNOSTIC PRODUCTS.

GMP (and hence this booklet) is all about the very special care and attention that is necessary to ensure that products like these are of the right QUALITY. GMP is vitally important in the manufacture of all types of product used in healthcare—drug products, diagnostics, medical devices, and so on. When it comes to sterile products, we have an additional quality that we must ensure. Quite simply, and obviously, we must ensure that our sterile products are, *in fact*, STERILE.

So, before we go any further, we need to be absolutely certain what we mean by the words "QUALITY" and "STERILE." Let's deal with "Quality" first.

"Quality" is one of those words that can have a lot of different meanings. Sometimes the word is used to mean "excellence" or "goodness." On the other hand, in a more technical sense, some people say that a thing is the right QUALITY when it meets (or complies with) a specification.

These uses of the word "QUALITY" are not wrong. It is just that there **are** different possible meanings. When we are talking about the manufacture of products like the ones listed above, we mean something that is both wider and more simple. We say:

QUALITY IS FITNESS FOR ITS INTENDED PURPOSE.

Now, as we know, a number of things are necessary before we can say that a product of the sort we are talking about is Fit for its Intended Purpose. For example, it must be:

- The Right Product (Obviously!).

- Of the Right Strength (where applicable).

- Free from any significant Contamination.

- In no way deteriorated, broken down, or damaged.

- In its proper container, correctly labeled, and properly sealed, so that it is protected against damage and contamination.

Now these things all apply to all drug (or pharmaceutical), medical, and similar products. Very great care, following the principles of Good Manufacturing Practice (GMP), is needed when making all these products, whether they are sterile or not. What makes STERILE products different, extra special even, is that they must be completely free from one particular type of contamination. That is, they must be free from contamination by living organisms (things like germs, "bugs," or microbes).

All the normal standards of GMP must apply, and these are outlined in the first booklet in this series: *Quality Rules—A Short Guide to Drug Products GMP*. BUT, on top of all that, there are additional "extra special" requirements that are necessary to ensure that one very important quality—STERILITY.

So, what does "STERILE" mean? Well, we have just hinted at its meaning. It does not just mean "super clean." It means the complete absence of living things. That is, no "germs" and things like that (the "proper" or better word for these is "microorganisms") in or on the product. Note: "*complete absence*." A thing cannot be "nearly sterile" or "almost sterile." There are no half measures—NO MICROORGANISMS. Period!

The process of making things sterile (that is, the process of removing or destroying microorganisms) is called "Sterilization." There are a number of different ways of doing this, and we will deal with some of these later.

Why do products of the sorts we listed above have to be sterile?

The most important reason is that there are great dangers of causing serious harm to patients if they are not.

When things are taken by mouth (for example tablets, capsules, syrups, etc.) the body has certain natural defenses against at least low levels of microbial contamination. (Although, of course, it is not a good idea that even these products should be contaminated with dangerous organisms.) Products required to be given in, or through, more sensitive areas must be sterile.

Injected products bypass the body's natural defenses against microorganisms, and the consequences of injecting even slightly contaminated products can be very serious. Injection of products contaminated with microorganisms **can cause, and has caused, death**. The same applies to things like devices, instruments, and implants that are intended to be inserted into blood vessels, muscles, or other parts of the body.

For the same reason, products intended for use in the eye (like drops, ointments, or lotions), for application to wounds, sores, or broken skin (like liquids, creams, ointments, or dressings), or used in operations to irrigate (wash out) body cavities or wounds must be sterile. It is also usually considered best that ear drops should be sterile, and some consider that nose drops should be sterile as well.

Before we finish this first section, we must deal with one more very important point. You remember that we mentioned that some people say that a product is the right quality when it meets (or complies with) a specification? You will also already know that this is an unsatisfactory and incomplete definition of "quality" when we are dealing with things like medicines, drug products, or medical devices. It is even more unsatisfactory when we are talking about STERILE medicines, pharmaceuticals, and devices. You see, in order to decide whether or not something meets a specification, we have to carry out tests. And this is where the big crunch comes.

The reality is that there is no test that will reliably confirm that a batch of sterile product is, in fact, sterile. Sure, there is a test called the Sterility Test. However, it is such a poor test that it would be perfectly possible for a batch of product to pass it, even if quite a lot of the containers or articles in the batch were contaminated with microorganisms. You must **never think that because a product has passed the sterility test, then it must be sterile.** It is even more dangerous to think that if errors have been made in manufacture and the product is partly contaminated, then the sterility test will be able to detect this. The chances are that it will NOT. Assurance of sterility can only be obtained by the utmost care and attention to detail at all stages in the manufacture of the product.

To sum up, important RULES to remember are:

1. **"Sterile" means "NO living things." In particular, it means no microorganisms (germs, bugs, and things like that).**

2. **Sterilization is the process of making something sterile, that is, destroying or removing all living things.**

3. **It is very difficult (for all practical purposes, we could say that it is impossible) to prove conclusively that every part, or unit, of every batch we make is sterile.**

4. **For this reason, EXTRA SPECIAL care, attention, and the highest standards of Good Manufacturing Practice are necessary.**

5. **Sterile products of the sort we are talking about are among the most difficult of all products to make properly. But if they are not made properly, they can be very dangerous indeed. They can KILL.**

The rest of this booklet is about this EXTRA SPECIAL CARE— about how we control contamination by microorganisms (and other things) and, finally, about how we sterilize our materials and products. But first we need to know something about "the enemy." That is, we need to know about the different types and sources of contamination.

2. TYPES OF CONTAMINATION

As we've already said, the most important thing about the manufacture of Sterile Products is the prevention, destruction, or removal of a form of contamination, that is, contamination by microorganisms. But in addition to these tiny living things, there are other sorts of contamination we have to keep out or remove as well.

We can classify the various possible forms of CONTAMINATION into two main types:

- LIVING (or VIABLE) contamination

and

- NONLIVING (or NONVIABLE) contamination.

Let us first talk a little more about those **living** forms of contamination.

Most people have heard of "germs," even if all that they know about them is that they are things that are small, and that they are probably nasty. Even that is not entirely true. Sure, "germs" are small (very small!) but, in everyday life, by no means are all of them nasty. In fact, although some of them are *very* nasty, others are useful to us.

Other words that mean more or less the same as "germs" are "Microbes" or "Microorganisms." Perhaps the best (and most "scientific") word to use is MICROORGANISMS. "Organisms" means "living things," and "micro" means "very small." So, "microorganisms" just means "very small living things." The advantage of the word "microorganism" is that we can use it to include things other than germs (or bacteria). Microorganisms include:

- BACTERIA ("GERMS"),

- MOLDS and FUNGI,

- YEASTS,

and

- VIRUSES.

Each of these different main groups of microorganisms includes many different types, species, or varieties.

Single microorganisms cannot be seen with the naked eye, but only with the aid of quite powerful microscopes. They are so small that it would take about a million of them to cover the head of a pin. However, we can see them (and their effects) when lots of them are growing together to form what we call a colony, or when, for example, they are growing on food, turning it rotten.

That's the problem with microorganisms. There can be many millions of them present on a surface, or in a liquid, without us having any idea that they are there. Think, for example, of a one-liter bottle of infusion fluid ("drip"). When made, it should look clear and bright. Even if only a few microorganisms are present at first, under the right conditions (that is, the right conditions for them), they could grow and multiply very rapidly. Yet, even if there are ONE MILLION microorganisms present in every ml. (and that would mean a billion in a liter bottle!), then only the very keenest eyesight can detect the very, very faint cloudiness caused in the liquid. For the average pair of eyes to be able to detect just a very faint "milkiness," Ten Million microorganisms would need to be present per ml. That is 10,000,000,000 (ten billion) in the whole bottle!!!

So, that's how small they are. We also said that they are LIV-ING things, and they certainly are. They GROW. . . . They FEED. . . . and they REPRODUCE themselves. Some can move about in liquids or on wet surfaces. Some respire, using the oxygen from the air like we do, but not all of them. In fact, some of them cannot grow at all in the presence of oxygen. On the other hand, most can survive without oxygen for quite a long time. But the three things that they ALL must have to grow and reproduce are MOISTURE, FOOD, and WARMTH.

Nevertheless, be warned! The lack of these three essentials will not necessarily KILL microorganisms. They just will not flourish, grow, and reproduce themselves without them. Many of them are great survivors under the most trying conditions, but if we remove moisture, food, and warmth (that is, keep things DRY, CLEAN, and COOL [or COLD]), we will at least have made a good step toward controlling the spread of microorganisms, even if we have not killed or completely removed them.

Another thing to remember is that even the most extreme cold does not kill them. It just keeps them under control. That is, it stops them growing and multiplying. But, even in a deep freezer, they stay alive. When things warm up, they get going again.

As for food—well, although some types (or species) are very fussy about what they will or will not feed on, microorganisms as a whole can use an amazing variety of substances for food. Obviously, they can live on things like meat, fruit, milk, bread, and jelly. Many are very happy feeding on just plain "muck." Some have been known to feed on the most unlikely things—like jet fuel and even disinfectants.

BACTERIA are single-celled organisms; although some species, particularly the ones called COCCI, tend to join up together to form pairs, chains, or bunches. These are called DIPLOCOCCI (pairs), STREPTOCOCCI (chains), and STAPHY-LOCOCCI (bunches).

(Note: "Cocci" is the plural. We talk of one coccus, or several cocci.)

Other sorts of bacteria include the rod-shaped BACILLI, some of which are covered in short hairs or "cilia," and some of which have long hairs, or "flagellae." One example of a Bacillus with flagellae is Listeria, some strains of which have been found in foods and can cause serious infections.

Other sorts of Bacteria are the comma-shaped VIBRIOS, and the wriggly- or spiral-shaped SPIROCHAETES.

(The drawings in Figure X on the next page give a rough idea of what some of these sorts of bacteria look like when highly magnified under a microscope.)

These are, however, just some of the main groups of Bacteria. As far as different SPECIES or varieties are concerned—well, there are many thousands of different species and varieties. Like all living things, they all have fairly complicated names, derived from the ancient Latin language.

Although it might seem that these names are a bit of a put-off, they do make sense. They are international; that is, they are standard and understood throughout the world.

The BAD effects of just a few bacteria and the diseases they cause are as follows:

(Now look, you don't need to remember these names. This is to give you an idea of the harm that some microorganisms can cause. In fact, if you want to, for now you could skip the next bit.)

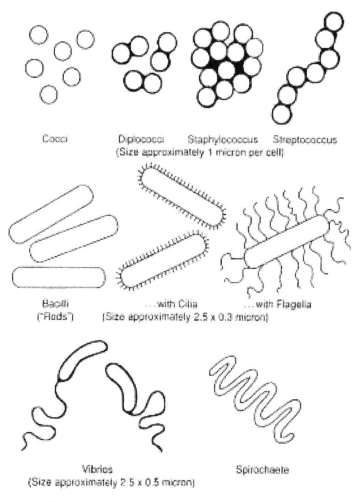

SOME TYPES OF BACTERIA—As seen under the Microscope

Cocci   Diplococci   Staphylococcus Streptococcus
(Size approximately 1 micron per cell)

Bacilli   ...with Cilia   ...with Flagella
("Rods") (Size approximately 2.5 x 0.3 micron)

Vibrios   Spirochaete
(Size approximately 2.5 x 0.5 micron)

Note: Drawings are not to scale. One micron = 1/1000 mm.

Figure X shows some types of bacteria, as seen under a microscope.

Bacteria	Disease
Staphylococcus aureus	boils, sties, impetigo, conjunctivitis (If transferred on to food, it can cause food poisoning)
Streptococcus pyogenes	tonsillitis, scarlet fever, rheumatic fever
Diplococcus pneumoniae	pneumonia, meningitis, peritonitis
Neisseria gonorrhoeae (a form of *coccus*)	gonorrhoea
Bacillus anthracis	anthrax
Bacillus cereus	food poisoning
Vibrio cholerae	cholera
Treponema pallidum (a *Spirochaete*)	syphilis

As for the number of individual bacteria that there are in the world, well there are so many billions of billions of them that it is just not possible to imagine. This is because, in conditions that are favorable (to them), they can reproduce themselves at an amazing rate.

Bacteria reproduce by the simple process of each individual dividing itself in half (a sort of multiplication by division). Under good conditions, that is, when they have moisture, food, and warmth, they can divide in this way about once every twenty minutes. So, in twenty minutes, one bacterium becomes two bacteria; in forty minutes, four; in an hour, eight;

and so on. How many do you think there will be in twelve hours? The answer is over two million million!

You will remember that we said that, in addition to BACTERIA, the other main sorts of microorganisms are MOLDS, YEASTS, and VIRUSES.

MOLDS are also called FUNGI. They come in many different shapes and sizes. They can look like a very fine network on a surface. They can also form larger structures like mushrooms, toadstools, and similar forms.

YEASTS are a form of mold. Under a microscope, they look rather like Bacteria, but are usually a little larger.

VIRUSES are perhaps the oddest form of microorganism (you could say that they are on the borderline between the living and the nonliving) and they can only grow inside another living cell. That is, they have no independent existence.

In addition to some of the bacteria, some molds, yeasts, and viruses can also cause illness, but by no means are all microorganisms harmful. In fact, in normal circumstances, the great majority of them are quite harmless. A number of them are very useful. For example, they are needed to make beer, wine, bread, cheese, and yogurt. Some live normally, and quite naturally, in our digestive tract. We provide them with shelter, food, warmth, and moisture. In return, some of them help us with our digestion. Others, living in the ground, break down dead plants and animals and, in this way, help to recycle nutrients in the soil.

But others are indeed BAD—bad for us, that is. As we have seen, some cause diseases, from the most minor illnesses to those that cause death. Others can spoil food, or other things like medicinal and cosmetic creams and lotions.

Even the ones that are normally harmless can be a danger if given to people who are already ill.

That is the reason why, as far as possible, microorganisms should be kept out of, and off of, drug products and medical devices of all types. Products that are intended to be INJECTED or used in the EYE, on OPEN WOUNDS, or inserted in BODY CAVITIES, TISSUES, or BLOOD VESSELS must be STERILE—that is, completely free from all living organisms. That is because even organisms that normally do not cause disease can be very dangerous if they exist in or on products which are intended to be injected or inserted into the body of a patient. People have been killed as a consequence of being injected with fluids that were contaminated with microorganisms of a type that normally do not cause disease.

You will remember that in addition to these living forms of contamination that we must keep out, remove, or destroy when we are making Sterile Products, we also have to protect our products against NONLIVING CONTAMINATION.

We can also classify this nonliving contamination into two main groups:

ACTIVE CONTAMINATION and INERT (or INACTIVE) CONTAMINATION.

By "Active," we mean chemically active, or having some activity when introduced into the human (or other animal) body. So, we can classify contamination overall, as follows:

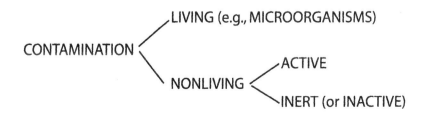

And even that is not the whole story, because there are still other special forms of contaminating substances that we must guard against. These are called PYROGENS, and we will talk about them shortly.

ACTIVE NONLIVING CONTAMINATION

It is easy to understand why Sterile Products must not be contaminated in this way. Here, we are talking about things like powder, dust, or crystals from other batches of product, or residues of other solutions, suspensions, or creams "left over" in containers, vessels, or equipment that have not been properly cleaned and dried. Many chemical substances can have very powerful effects, even in very small amounts, when they enter the human body. The effect can be very serious when they are swallowed. It can be a lot worse if they are injected. So, it is obvious that this sort of contamination must not be allowed to happen to sterile products. The air in rooms used for Sterile Products manufacture, and all floors, walls, surfaces, equipment, vessels, containers, and so on must be kept free of active chemical contaminants in order to prevent them getting on or in the product being manufactured. Steps need to be taken, too, to prevent chemical contamination from the dust on the clothes and shoes of people who have been using or weighing bulk chemical substances.

All this is fairly obvious. Perhaps not quite so obvious is the significance of:

INERT NONLIVING CONTAMINATION

What we are talking about here are nonactive little bits, fibers, particles, and things like that. This is often called "PARTICU-LATE CONTAMINATION," or just "PARTICULATES." Don't get confused. It is really very simple. "Particles," "Particulate Contamination," and "Particulates" all mean the same thing—little bits of things floating about in the air or in liquids, or deposited on surfaces.

The list of such things is almost endless—atmospheric and house dust, fine soil, sand, ash, smoke, dandruff, skin flakes, pollen, fibers (from natural and artificial textiles or from paper), flaking paint, powdering plaster or masonry, metal particles from moving machine parts or from drilled or ground metals, rubber or composition particles from belt drives in machines, and so on.

There has been a lot of discussion and argument over the dangers (or otherwise) of fine particles when they are injected or inserted into the body. Clearly we do not want to have hard particles in eye drops, and it is well known that excessive inhalation of a wide range of dusts causes serious lung problems. Surprisingly, some scientists have argued that the injection of particles is not all that dangerous. On the other hand, others claim that there are hazards, and that injected particles can block small blood vessels, or pass to the lungs and block the fine bronchial tubes, or lodge in the liver and causes damage, and so on. So, in spite of some of the arguments, it is considered necessary to control the level of particles in injections (and other Sterile Products). Pharmacopoeias (the official books that set standards for medicines and things like that—a fine example is *The United States Pharmacopoeia* or USP) specify the levels that are permitted for particles in certain injections and other Sterile Products. This, in turn, means controlling the numbers of particles in the rooms (in the air and on surfaces) in which Sterile Products are made.

There is another very good reason for keeping down contamination by these inert PARTICLES. It is that most airborne bacteria and other microorganisms do not just float around in the air on their own. They are usually attached to particles. So, if we control the level of particles generally, we have made one good step towards controlling the level of microorganisms.

PYROGENS

As we have said, there is another form of possible dangerous contamination. Although it is NONLIVING, it is, in fact, produced by the living organisms that may be present, for example, in water or in a solution. This contamination may also be present on the surfaces of containers, vessels, instruments, devices, and other materials that have been in contact with fluids containing this form of contamination, or that have been left wet so that microorganisms can develop. These contaminants are called PYROGENS (another expression you may hear that means more-or-less the same thing is "BACTERIAL ENDOTOXINS"). Pyrogens are quite complex chemical compounds that are produced by living and growing microorganisms in the course of their normal life processes. When injected or otherwise inserted into people (or into any other animals), they can cause quite high rises in body temperature (the word "Pyro-gen" means "giving rise to heat"), plus other highly undesirable effects.

A dangerous increase in temperature is the last thing we want to happen to a patient who is already ill, and since most sterilization processes do not necessarily remove or destroy pyrogens, it is very important that we guard against the development and growth of microorganisms, and the consequent formation of pyrogens. We CANNOT rely just on the sterilization process itself to ensure that the product is both sterile AND free from pyrogens. Many sterilization processes, although they will destroy the microorganisms, may not destroy the pyrogens present. Very careful control over the entire manufacturing cycle is essential to ensure that pyrogen-producing organisms are excluded, or at least kept to a minimum, *throughout* the process.

To sum up on Types of Contamination:

1. **There are two main types of contamination—LIVING and NONLIVING.**

2. **When making Sterile Products, our concern is particularly with preventing, removing, or destroying very small living things—MICROORGANISMS, that is, things like Bacteria (germs), Molds, Yeasts, and Viruses.**

3. There are many millions of millions of these microorganisms. They can reproduce themselves and spread very rapidly.

4. Some microorganisms are very dangerous to us. Others can be quite harmless or even useful, in some circumstances. ALL OF THEM MUST BE KEPT AWAY OR REMOVED FROM STERILE PRODUCTS.

5. NONLIVING contamination, whether it is an active chemical substance, or just inactive dust, powder, or fibers, must be kept out of, or off of, Sterile Products.

6. Living microorganisms can produce dangerous PYROGENS. These must not be allowed to develop in, or on, Sterile Products.

3. SOURCES OF CONTAMINATION

We have already talked about the way some forms of contamination can arise. Let us now take a look at some of these sources of contamination in a little more detail.

SOURCES OF NONLIVING CONTAMINATION

CONTAMINATION by ACTIVE CHEMICAL substances can be caused by dust and powder in the air, or that has settled on surfaces, vessels, or equipment. It can also arise from residues ("left overs") in or on containers, vessels, and equipment that have been used for other products or materials and that have not been properly cleaned. Other possible sources include traces of materials that have been used for cleaning and disinfection.

There are many possible sources of what we called INERT NONLIVING CONTAMINATION (or "Particulate Contamination"). For example:

- **Buildings**—Unsealed stonework, brick, mortar, plaster, flaking paint, and things like that.

- **Materials**—Ingredients that might not be highly active in themselves can nevertheless be a big source of highly undesirable particles.

- **Equipment**—Dirty equipment, moving machine parts, and belt drives.

What we could call "the General Environment" can deposit a wide range of contaminants—dust, dirt, soil, sand, smoke, ash, and things like that.

Containers, Packages, Paper, and Cardboard can all produce enormous amounts of fibrous contamination.

Filtered air supplies to the rooms in which Sterile Products are manufactured, although intended to reduce particulate contamination, can have the reverse effect if the filters are damaged, or if the system is not properly maintained.

So you see there is a very wide range of possible sources of the NONLIVING CONTAMINATION from which our Sterile Products must be protected. BUT (and it is a very important "BUT"):

the biggest source of contamination is usually **PEOPLE AND THEIR CLOTHING.**

By the use of what we call CLEAN ROOMS, we can achieve quite a high level of control over particles. Put people in a room, and it is a different story. Up to 80 percent of the particulate contamination in Clean Rooms is due to people.

We all shed thousands of millions of dead skin cells and fragments per day. This amounts to a total weight of somewhere between five and fifteen grams per day of tiny bits and pieces that fall off us. The more we move, and the more vigorously that we move, the greater the shedding becomes. We shed three or four times more particles when we move about than when we are at rest. Depending on the type of cloth, we also disperse large numbers of fibers from our clothing. This amount also increases as we move about.

We shed something like 1,000 bacteria-carrying particles per minute. People are, indeed, a major source of both living and nonliving contamination. That is why one of the main concerns in Sterile Products manufacture is to protect the products being made from the people who are making them. And that brings us to the sources of LIVING CONTAMINATION, that is, those microorganisms we have already talked about.

SOURCES OF MICROORGANISMS

Where do microorganisms come from?

Well the simple answer is that, like all other organisms (including people), they don't just "happen." They come from "parent" microorganisms. The big difference is, of course, that in favorable conditions they multiply so much more rapidly than, for example, we do.

Microorganisms are almost everywhere. Some have managed to flourish in strong acids, some in hot springs, and some even in certain disinfectants. They are found, by the millions, in or on:

- **The environment around us**. That is, in the air (indoors and out), on the ground, in the soil, on walls, floors, and surfaces generally—almost everywhere.

- **Water**. They exist in the water from the faucet, in rivers, seas, and lakes; in puddles, on wet surfaces and wet floors; and in damp surfaces of containers and equipment that have not been properly dried. In general, bacteria will be found in all water, whether it is in large quantities or just light surface films, except water that has been specially sterilized and sealed against any recontamination.

- **The raw materials** we use for making products.

- **The containers and closures** we use for packaging our products.

All these are sources of contamination that we can do something about. It is not always easy, but we can. There is the other source of contamination, and it is a major one, which is rather more difficult to deal with. That is PEOPLE. In spite of increasing automation, it is still necessary to involve people in the manufacture of Sterile Products, and we cannot sterilize people (in the microbiological sense), or treat them with strong disinfectants, or eliminate them altogether.

PEOPLE AS A SOURCE OF CONTAMINATION

People (that is, us) are a major, indeed perhaps the biggest, source of contamination by microorganisms. They live on us, and inside us. They live on our skin surfaces, particularly in hair and beards and in moist, hairy parts generally, and they live in our digestive tract.

We shed bacteria-carrying particles by the million, all the time, particularly from our:

- Skin,

- Hair,

- Beard,

- Digestive Tract,

- Saliva,

- Nose,

- Mouth,

and

- Throat.

We blow them out (MILLIONS of them!) when we cough, sneeze, and splutter—even when we just breathe, and even more when we talk, shout, sing, or whistle.

We become particularly dangerous if we have opens wounds, cuts, or grazes, or if we have respiratory infections (like coughs, colds, and bronchitis) or digestive tract infections (diarrhea, enteritis, and so on).

Anyone suffering from even minor surface injuries, or from any infections (like those above, or any others), must report them to their supervisor.

It is, of course, important that all persons working on all drug and similar products should maintain high standards of personal cleanliness and hygiene—clean skin, clean hands, clean hair, clean bodies, and clean clothes. This is even more important when Sterile Products are being manufactured.

Although there should never be any direct contact between hands and products (except when they are in sealed containers), hands must always be kept clean and, of course, thoroughly washed and dried after going to the bathroom.

Bacteria can spread from people to people, and from people to things, in a variety of ways, including coughing, sneezing, scratching, fingering nose, shaking hands, and so on.

Since we cannot entirely eliminate the microorganisms that are in and on us, we must take special care to protect the products that we are making from them.

Key points to remember about Sources of Contamination are:

1. **There are very many possible sources of the different forms of contamination.**

2. **Particular problems arise from dusty, dirty premises, from uncleaned or wet equipment and containers, from the air, and from water.**

3. **The biggest and most difficult problem, however, is usually the contamination caused by people, who can be a major source of contamination by both particles and microorganisms.**

A GOLDEN RULE in making Sterile Products is: Always be on the lookout for possible contamination, and guard against it.

4. CONTROL OF CONTAMINATION—CLEAN ROOMS

Now that we know something about the different sorts of contamination, and where it all can come from, we can talk a little about the sort of things we must do to keep contamination under control and, ultimately, to eliminate it.

When making a Sterile Product, one of our main aims is to eliminate completely any microorganisms in or on the product by killing them or removing them in some other way. This total destruction or removal of organisms is called STERILIZATION, and in the manufacture of a Sterile Product, there will, at some stage or other, be one or more sterilization process(es). In addition to the product itself, things like water (and other solvents), containers, mixing vessels, equipment, and pipelines may all need to be sterilized.

We will be talking about different methods of sterilization later, but before we do so, there are some more very important things to remember.

If we want to be absolutely sure of sterilizing something, we must not just think that a normal sterilization process will sterilize anything, no matter how heavily contaminated it is. If we were to set our product alight and burn it all to ash, we could be pretty sure that we had killed all the organisms present, but we would then have no product! Sterilization processes are usually rather less drastic than that. So the chances of sterilizing something that is only lightly contaminated are much greater than if we attempted to sterilize something that was very heavily loaded with microorganisms like, say, raw sewage. The aim is always to present to the actual sterilization process a product or material which is as microbiologically "clean" as possible. To put it another way, we say that, in order to present a low challenge to the sterilization process, the product or material to be sterilized should have a low *bioburden*. ("Bioburden" is a word that simply means the amount of microorganisms in, or on, the product or material.) This is another example of that need for extra special care all along the line.

It is also important to remember that sterilization processes are not necessarily designed to remove or destroy all the other forms of contamination we have mentioned. A product or material could be sterile, and yet still be contaminated with dangerous levels of active chemical substances, particles, or pyrogens. Certainly, if pyrogen levels are to be kept low, microbial contamination must be kept under strict control.

So that is why it is important to take great care to control or keep out all forms of contamination before we even get to the stage of sterilizing the product. Of course, once something has been sterilized, it is essential to ensure that it does not become recontaminated. If a product is first sealed in its final container and *then* sterilized (this is called "Terminal Sterilization"), there should be no further risk of recontamination, at least until the container is opened. However, if the product is sterilized *before* it is filled (or packed) and sealed in its final container, then very great care is necessary to prevent recontamination after the sterilization process. But we are jumping ahead! We must first talk about keeping contamination under control, before and after sterilization.

CLEAN ROOMS

One obvious way to control contamination of products is to work in an especially clean environment. That is, in rooms where contamination of all types—in the air, on walls, floors, and all surfaces—is maintained and controlled at a really low level. That is why so much of the manufacture of Sterile Products, and certainly all those stages where the product or its container could be exposed to contamination, is carried out in Clean Rooms.

"CLEAN ROOM" in this special sense does **not** just mean a room that is clean. It means a room in which there is careful control, within defined limits, of the quality (or clean-ness) of the air inside that room. This clean-ness is defined in terms of the numbers of particles that are permitted per cubic foot (or per cubic meter) of air in the room. In a Clean Room, the numbers of particles in the air are much lower (in the case of the higher Classes of Clean Room, very much lower) than in an ordinary room. So, in a high Class Clean Room the air is very much cleaner than in the cleanest of ordinary rooms. This is achieved by forcing air into the room, under pressure, through air filters.

In most cases (there are some exceptions), in a Clean Room used for the manufacture of Sterile Products, the air pressure in the Room is kept higher than in the "world" or factory outside. Furthermore, the pressure has to be highest where the product may be exposed (and is therefore at risk from contamination), with the air pressure becoming successively lower in the various other rooms that, together, form the overall Sterile Manufacturing area, or "Suite." The aim is that Sterile Manufacturing areas will always be flushed by filtered clean air in a way designed to sweep contamination away from the product or the materials used in making it. The exceptions we mentioned include rooms where penicillins and live vaccines are handled, where it is important to prevent the spread of such materials from the room. In all cases, it is very important that checks are constantly made to ensure that Clean Room air pressures are maintained at the levels specified and that the air flows in the directions intended. This is done by the use of various air pressure measuring devices (called manometers) and by other techniques.

Throughout the world, there are a number of official published Standards for Clean Rooms that define the number and sizes of particles permitted in Clean Rooms of different Classes. Standards for Clean Rooms were originally devised for use in the microelectronic and aerospace industries, where it is important to protect tiny electronic components from even the finest particles. Later, the pharmaceutical and related industries adopted similar Clean Room standards for Sterile Products Manufacture, and added to them permissible limits for the numbers of microorganisms in the air.

The first widely accepted Clean Room Standard was the US Federal Standard 209. It was published in the 1960s, and has gone through a number of revisions over the years. The latest version is Federal Standard 209E. The basic idea, however, has remained the same. Clean Rooms are classified according to the maximum number of particles (of a size 0.5 microns or more) permitted per cubic foot of air. From our perspective, the important Clean Room Classes are Class 100, Class 10,000 and Class 100,000. That means that, for example, in a Class 100 Clean Room, no more than 100 particles (of a size 0.5 microns or more) are permitted per cubic foot of air.

A *micron* (or more correctly, a *micrometer*) is 1/1000th (0.001) of a millimeter, or one millionth of a meter.

(If you would like to know a little more about the classification of Clean Rooms, you can find some more information in the Appendix at the end of this booklet.)

The internal surface finishes of a Clean Room are also very important. The surfaces of all floors, walls, and ceilings must be hard, smooth, impervious (nonporous), and unbroken (that is, no cracks, holes, or other damage). There are three good reasons for this:

1. To prevent the shedding of particles that could come from brick or plaster.

2. To prevent the accumulation of dust and dirt—AND OF MICROORGANISMS—on rough or broken surfaces.

3. To permit easy and repeated cleaning and disinfection.

There should be no uncleanable gaps, cracks, holes, corners, surfaces, pipes, ducts, or fittings that could harbor dust, dirt, and microorganisms.

Access to Clean Rooms must be carefully controlled, and that applies to both people and things—things like materials, equipment, and apparatus. Access to (and exit from) Clean Rooms should only be through AIR LOCKS. An Air Lock is an enclosed space with a door at each end that is placed between rooms (for example, two different Class Clean Rooms) in order to control the air flow between the rooms when they need to be entered. It is usual to arrange, by some device or warning system, that both doors cannot be open at the same time. To have both the doors open at the same time would defeat the whole object of the air lock.

Air Locks may be intended either for the passage of people or of materials. The Changing Rooms through which people enter and exit from Clean Rooms, putting on or taking off their special Clean Room clothing as they go, could be considered elaborate forms of Air Locks.

In addition to AIR LOCKS and CHANGING ROOMS, there are a number of other important features of Clean Rooms that you are likely to come across. For example:

PASS-THROUGH HATCH: This is a sort of mini-Air Lock, inserted in a wall between two different rooms, usually at bench height. It serves the same purpose as an Air Lock, and is usually used for the passage of materials or equipment. Again, the two doors should not be opened (or openable) at the same time.

DOUBLE-ENDED STERILIZER: This is a sterilizer that has a door at each end. When inserted through a Clean Room wall, it means that items can be loaded into the sterilizer on one side of the wall, and (following sterilization) be taken out on the other. This has two main advantages—it guards against the contamination of a Clean Room that could happen if goods were transported in or out by other means, and it helps to pre-vent mix-ups between sterilized and unsterilized materials.

STERILIZING TUNNEL: This is an enclosed conveyor system on which, for example, ampules and vials can be conveyed into a filling room while (during their journey through the tun-nel) they are subjected to sufficient heat to sterilize them and to destroy any pyrogens.

CONTAINED WORKSTATIONS: These are small, entirely or partly enclosed working areas within a Clean Room with their own filtered air supply. They are intended to provide extra-special protection against contamination for products or materials. The air supply is usually "unidirectional," that is, it flows only in one direction, with (if it is not disturbed) a minimum of turbulence. These workstations are often called "Laminar Air Flow" (LAF) hoods or cabinets.

This unidirectional or Laminar Flow effect is achieved by the air being forced through special High Efficiency ("HEPA") filters so that it passes, in just one direction, over the material or product that is in need of special protection, sweeping away (and keeping away) any potential microbial or other contamination. The airflow may be either vertical or horizontal.

There is a special way of working at, or under, a Laminar Flow Cabinet or "Hood," and we will be talking about that later.

It is, of course, no use designing, building, and equipping Clean Rooms, and then just letting things slip, without regularly checking that everything remains up to standard as far as contamination control is concerned. Air pressures and flows must be continually monitored. The quality of the air and surfaces within the rooms must also be checked regularly, using such things as total particle counters, air samplers (for viable organisms), "settle slates" (petri dishes of nutrient jelly to check microbial "fallout"), surface swabs, and contact plates.

Just one other point about the air in these rooms. We must not forget that there are people working in them, so there needs to be heating/cooling of all this high quality air to ensure the right level of comfort, particularly for people clothed in the special garments, which can make them hot. It is important that operators do not get too warm, because the more we sweat, the more particles and organisms we shed. And that brings us to the final important point of this section. In a well-designed, well-built, well-maintained, and well-controlled Clean Room, we can achieve a very high level of contamination control. There is one big problem. PEOPLE. People have to work in Clean Rooms. They have to get in and out of them. And as we know, people are a very serious source of potential contamination. We will deal with this in the next section.

Sumary on Clean Rooms:

1. A number of stages in Sterile Product manufacture are carried out in Clean Rooms.

2. The term "Clean Room" has a special meaning in Sterile Product manufacture. It is not just a room that is clean.

3. A Clean Room is a room in which the air is supplied, under pressure, through special filters designed to keep any microorganisms and other particles in the air down to defined low levels.

4. There are different Classes of Clean Rooms. The Class that is required depends on the type of work that is done in the Room.

5. The surfaces of all floors, walls, ceilings, fittings, work-tops, etc. in a Clean Room must be hard, smooth, impervious (nonporous), and unbroken, so as to prevent the shedding of particles, to prevent the accumulation of dust, dirt, and microorganisms, and to permit easy and repeated cleaning and disinfection.

6. There must be no uncleanable gaps, cracks, holes, corners, surfaces, pipes, ducts, fittings, and so on that could harbor dust, dirt, and microorganisms.

7. Access to Clean Rooms must be carefully controlled, and that applies to both people and things, like materials, equipment, and apparatus. Access to (and exit from) Clean Rooms should only be through AIR LOCKS.

8. Special Air Locks are also formed by the Changing Rooms through which people enter and exit from Clean Rooms, putting on or taking off their special Clean Room clothing as they go.

5. CONTROL OF CONTAMINATION—PEOPLE

As we have said already, PEOPLE are the biggest contamination hazard to Clean Rooms and to products, because of both the microorganisms and the nonviable particles that we shed. We can sterilize equipment, and we can filter air, but we cannot sterilize or filter people!

So, it is very important that the people who are going to enter and work in sterile manufacturing areas should be selected carefully for the job. They must behave in a specially well-disciplined way and must strictly follow official written procedures.

Before they even *think* of entering a sterile manufacturing area, these people must:

- Have high standards of personal hygiene;

- Keep their body, hair, and clothing (under and outer) clean;

and

- Not be suffering from any disease or condition that could result in more-than-normal shedding and dispersal of microorganisms or nonviable particles.

It is also a good general rule that it is best to have as few people in a Clean Room as possible.

Let us take a look at some of these points in a bit more detail.

It must be obvious that people who work in Clean Rooms should keep themselves and their clothes very clean. They should bathe or shower, and wash their hair regularly. They should take action against excessive dandruff.

Some people, because of some physical or nervous condition, are just not suited to work in Clean Rooms. These include folks who:

- Have chronic skin, respiratory, or digestive tract diseases;

- Have allergies to the synthetic fabrics used in Clean Room clothing;

- Are abnormally high shedders of skin flakes or dandruff;

- Have nervous conditions resulting in excessive itching and scratching;

or who

- Suffer from claustrophobia (that is, they cannot bear to be in confined spaces—and Clean Rooms are often somewhat confined).

People who suffer from these sorts of condition must have our sympathy. They can probably do a great job elsewhere. It is just that a Clean Room is not the place for them. Even people working in sterile products manufacturing areas who do not have these sort of problems regularly or permanently *must* report it to their boss if they have such things as:

- coughs, colds, runny noses;

- lung, digestive tract, or skin infections;

- wounds, cuts, or grazes;

or

- sunburn, leading to peeling and flaking of skin.

It really is important that Clean Room workers report it if they have any of these conditions. They can then, as necessary, be temporarily assigned to other tasks where their condition is unlikely to cause harm.

There are a few more basic requirements for people entering and working in Clean Rooms. They should:

- NOT wear jewelry or wristwatches,

- NOT wear makeup or nail polish,

and

- Keep their fingernails short, as well as clean.

Makeup can flake off and create particles, and so can nail polish. Things like jewelry and wristwatches harbor dirt, particles, and sweat on, in, and under them. (Try feeling under your wristwatch on a warm day.) They can also cause excessive shedding of skin particles, due to rubbing against the skin. Some regulatory authorities consider that plain gold, or other precious metal, wedding rings are acceptable when worn under gloves. Others consider that the wearing of any sort of ring in a Clean Room is unacceptable.

So—those are some of the special requirements for people who work in Clean Rooms. We will now take a look at how people get in and out of these rooms, and what they should and should not do when they are in them.

ENTRY TO CLEAN ROOMS

Clean Rooms must only be entered by persons authorized to do so, and through the special Changing Rooms provided.

In the changing rooms, personnel change from their regular factory overalls into special Clean Room protective garments.

These garments are themselves clean, and in Class 100 Clean Rooms, where sterilized products or materials may be exposed (that is, in what are called "Aseptic Processing Areas"), they must also be sterile.

Outdoor clothing should not be taken into changing rooms. It should have been left behind when and where the operators put on their regular factory overalls.

The special clothing provided must always be worn when working in Clean Rooms, and must not be worn outside the Clean Room or changing room.

CHANGING PROCEDURES

The purpose of the protective clothing worn in a Clean Room is to protect the room environment AND THE PRODUCT from the particles, fibers, and microorganisms shed by the operator wearing it. It is also important that the protective garment itself should shed very few particles or fibers. These garments are specially designed and made to achieve these objectives. Most commonly, they are one- or two-piece pantsuits, fitting closely at wrists and ankles, and with high necks. Headwear must totally enclose the hair and beard or mustache, if the operator has one. Powder-free rubber or plastic gloves are worn, with the sleeves of the suit tucked securely inside the gloves. Footwear should totally enclose the feet and ankles, and the pants bottoms should be tucked inside the footwear. Masks should cover nose and mouth. The result should be that the only exposed parts of the body are the eyes, and even these may be required to be covered by goggles.

That was a very general outline of Clean Room garments. They vary in form and detail from one company to another, and in accordance with the type of process being performed. The important thing is that the garments must be worn properly and put on carefully, following the company's written CHANGING PROCEDURE. This will include details of hand and arm washing, as well as instructions for changing into the protective garments. The level of stripping-off before putting these on will depend on the nature of the product and the process, but certainly any bulky or fluffy clothing should be removed.

The important RULES to remember are that:

- **The written Changing Procedure *must* be followed, EXACTLY.**

- **When changing, the Clean Room garments must be put on properly, taking care to avoid contaminating the outside of them as you do it.**

A good example of this last point is the use of the "step-over" (or "sit-over") bench (or barrier) when changing footwear. While sitting on the bench, with both feet on the "dirty side," a shoe is first removed from one foot, leaving the shoe on the dirty side. The Clean Room footwear is then put on this first foot, as it is swung over the bench and placed down on the floor of the clean side. The first foot is now on the clean side of the barrier, while the other remains on the dirty side. The process is now repeated with the second foot. This is easier to demonstrate than to describe. If it is done properly, the operator now has both feet (in Clean Room footwear) on the floor of the clean side, and has left two dirty shoes on the dirty side.

NOTHING that could cause contamination should be taken into a Clean Room, and that includes things like food, drink, candy, tissues, combs, and anything made from paper or cardboard materials.

EXIT *from* a Clean room should only be through a changing room, where the special Clean Room clothing is removed. This too should be done following the official written procedure.

ACTIVITIES IN CLEAN ROOMS

It is VITAL to remember that working in a Clean Room is different from other kinds of work activity. In addition to all the things we have already said about hygiene, health, and clothing, people in Clean Rooms must also behave in a special way. You see, although we all shed a lot of particles and microorganisms even when just sitting still, the rate and amount of shedding increases enormously when we move about. The more active we are, the more we shed. So this is one area of work where there are *no* prizes for rushing about or superfast working! All movements should be made at a steady, controlled rate.

A special case is working at, or under, Laminar Air Flow cabinet or hood—those "contained workstations" we talked about earlier. When working at, or under, Laminar Air Flow, it is important to ensure that:

- Nothing is placed between the face of the air filter and the object, material, or product that is being handled and that needs to be protected. (This would disturb the smoothly sweeping flow of unidirectional air that is intended to keep vital areas clean.)

- The operator always works downstream from the air filter face, and does not let hands or arms come between the item that is being protected and the filter. (It makes no sense to blow contamination from an operator on to a product.)

In all types of Clean Rooms, if something falls to the floor, it is usually best to leave it there until the room has a general cleanup—unless, of course, it would be dangerous to leave the object on the floor.

It is important always to remember that, having got an operator successfully through a changing room routine, "scrubbed up" and properly dressed in the protective garment, much now depends on how he or she behaves in the Clean Room. With this in mind, and recalling the other things we have said about people in Clean Rooms, we can now sum up with some important:

RULES ABOUT ENTERING AND WORKING IN CLEAN ROOMS

1. Keep body, hair, face, hands, and fingernails clean—really CLEAN.

2. Report any illnesses, cuts or grazes, and any respiratory, digestive tract, or skin infections.

3. Follow the written Changing and Washup procedures EXACTLY.

4. Check that your protective clothing is worn correctly.

5. Do not wear cosmetics, jewelry, or wristwatches.

6. Leave all personal items (wallets, purses, coins, keys, watches, tissues, combs, and so on) in the changing room.

7. Do not take papers, documents, or paper materials into a Clean Room, unless these have been specifically approved. (Paper, cardboard, and similar materials are great shedders of particles and fibers.)

8. No eating, chewing, drinking, or smoking.

9. Always move about gently and steadily.

10. Do NOT move vigorously. NO fooling around, singing, or whistling.

11. Keep talking to an absolute minimum.

12. Avoid coughing or sneezing. If these things are unavoidable, leave the Clean Room. (We spray a lot of fine drops and microbes about when we talk, sing, whistle, cough, sneeze, or splutter.)

13. Do not touch other operators.

14. Avoid scratching or touching nose or mouth, and rubbing hands.

15. Regularly disinfect gloves, as instructed.

16. Always check for worn or damaged garments and torn gloves, and change them as necessary. (Even a pinhole in a glove could have disastrous consequences for a patient.)

17. Keep garments fully fastened up. Do not unfasten or loosen them.

18. Unless there is a special hazard involved, do not pick up items from the floor.

You see, working on the manufacture of Sterile Products does require *very disciplined behavior.* Nobody has ever said that making Sterile Products is easy, and all these things are necessary to ensure the safety of patients.

6. CONTROL OF CONTAMINATION—CLEANING AND DISINFECTION

So far we have talked about the importance of Clean Rooms and the influence of People in the control of contamination. We are now going to discuss two other factors that are important in contamination control—CLEANING and DISINFECTION.

Cleaning is quite simply the removal of dust, dirt, debris, residues, and so on. This dirt (by definition, dirt is stuff in the wrong place) can arise from a number of sources, including:

- Airborn dust, dirt, and particles;

- Particles, fibers, hairs, and exudates shed by humans;

- Spillages and breakages;

- Particles from friction in machines;

- Oil and grease from lubricated moving parts;

- Residues from previous products;

and

- Just plain dirt. (It is one of the Fundamental Laws of Science that things that are not regularly cleaned get dirty!)

For obvious reasons, areas, surfaces, and equipment in and on which we make sterile products must be kept clean. We must not let dirt, and the microbes that it can harbor, get into or onto our products. But there is another good reason for regularly and scrupulously cleaning away this dirt.

Floors, walls, ceilings, and work surfaces need to be regularly disinfected—and here's the point. Disinfectants can be inactivated by dirt, and dirt (particularly oily or greasy films, and protein-like matter) can also protect microorganisms against the action of disinfectants. So, before we DISINFECT, it is important that first we CLEAN.

Where gross amounts of dirt are present, it may be first necessary to remove most of it by scraping or scrubbing. Then, surfaces can be cleaned by the application of a cleaning agent, followed by rinsing. In most normal circumstances, all that is needed for the cleaning of floors, walls, and work surfaces is clean water with the addition of detergent, followed by a clean water rinse. The quality of the water used will depend on the nature of the operations carried out on, or near, the surfaces in question. Obviously, it must be microbiologically clean, and it may be appropriate for at least the final rinse water to be of high quality "Water for Injection" standard. (We will deal with the various grades of water in the next section.)

Manufacturing tanks, pipelines, and associated equipment need also to be cleaned and rinsed after use, and before any sterilization that may be necessary. This may be done by simple manual methods, but a more modern technique is called "CLEAN IN PLACE" or CIP. Here, cleaning is accomplished by automatically pumping cleaning agents and rinsing liquids, under pressure, around the entire system, without necessarily dismantling it.

DISINFECTION

A DISINFECTANT is a chemical substance, or combination of substances, that, when applied to surfaces, will kill microorganisms, with the exception of some bacterial spores. You remember that "sterilization" means the destruction or removal of all microorganisms, and indeed of all organisms generally? When we sterilize something, if we do it properly, we destroy (or remove) all life. A DISINFECTANT is something that cannot quite achieve that. We cannot be certain that, by use of chemical solutions alone, we can destroy all living organisms, particularly bacterial spores. We just do not have suitable chemicals available.

However, while we are aiming at producing products that are sterile, our aim with walls, floors, ceilings, and work surfaces is not necessarily that they should be sterile. Our aim usually is that they should be as clean as possible, and with any microbiological contamination kept to a minimum. We can, and usually do, manage this by keeping surfaces clean and disinfected.

(You may, by the way, hear other words that mean the same sort of thing as "DISINFECTANT"—words like "Germicide," "Bactericide," and "Biocide." There is a possibility of confusion here, because these words mean different things to different people. It's best to stick to "Disinfectant." Another word, "Antiseptic," means a milder substance that can, for example, be used on skin surfaces and wounds to control or prevent infection without harming the patient. Even here, some people confuse antiseptics with disinfectants.)

Types of Disinfectants

Quite a wide range of substances are used as disinfectants. They may be single substances, like alcohol or phenols, and there are a number of commercially available mixtures. It is usually best not to try to make your own mixtures. It could be dangerous, and some disinfectants can neutralize each other's activity.

Disinfecting agents vary in the range of their activity and in the concentrations at which they are effective. All have their own special advantages. They also have some disadvantages. (For example, alcohols are flammable, phenols and chlorine compounds can be dangerous and corrosive, iodine compounds can stain some surfaces, and so on.)

Disinfectants should always be used in accordance with instructions (as given either in the supplier's literature, or in company procedures) and at the right dilution. Dilutions of disinfectants should not be stored unless they are sterilized. Otherwise, dilutions should be made up freshly each time they are needed. (It is a fact that some microorganisms can grow in dilute disinfectants.)

Another "traditional" method of disinfecting Clean Rooms is by fumigating or "gassing," usually with formaldehyde gas, although this can present problems due to the unpleasant, choking, and toxic nature of the gas. An alternative is hydrogen peroxide vapor.

Rotation of Disinfectants

Many Sterile Product Manufacturers use different disinfectants over a period of time, on an alternating, or rotating, basis. The reasoning behind this is to prevent the development of disinfectant-resistant strains of microorganisms. Although there have been some arguments about it, alternation of disinfectants remains a recommendation of a number of experts and regulatory bodies.

CLEANING AND DISINFECTION IN PROCESSING AREAS

Routine cleaning and disinfection in Clean Rooms and other processing areas should be regularly carried out in accordance with an established program, following a standard written procedure. That is, cleaning and disinfection is NOT something to be done only when it seems like a good idea or when there is some spare time.

Not surprisingly, written programs and procedures will vary in detail from manufacturer to manufacturer, and in accordance with the type of product being manufactured. We can, however, set out some important general:

RULES ABOUT CLEANING AND DISINFECTION

1. The written program and procedure must always be followed—EXACTLY.

2. It is necessary to CLEAN thoroughly first, before disinfecting.

3. It is important to ensure that, in the cleaning and disinfecting process, we do not in fact create more contamination.

4. All cleaning and disinfecting agents and materials should themselves be clean and not shed fibers or particles. (You cannot CLEAN with muddy water and dirty, hairy cloths.)

5. Cleaning implements and wiping cloths, having been applied to a surface, should not be rewetted by direct return to the container of cleaning or disinfecting agent, but first rinsed (and squeezed out) in a second bucket of clean water.

6. Nonshedding materials should be used for wiping surfaces, and dry, dust-creating brushes should not be used. If it is necessary to remove significant quantities of powdery materials, then wet or vacuum methods are preferable.

7. All cleaning and disinfection of a room should start at the part of the room furthest from the entrance, otherwise there is a danger of the cleaner "painting himself into a corner," and having to cross the cleaned area in order to get out.

8. When cleaning walls and other vertical surfaces, work should always start at the top and work down—again, to avoid recontamination of parts already cleaned or disinfected.

9. It is vital that the right cleaning and disinfecting agents are used, in the right dilutions, as directed in the company's written procedure. Remember, dilutions of disinfectants

should be made up fresh, in clean containers. They should not be stored for later use unless they are sterilized.

10. All cleaning equipment and implements must themselves be thoroughly cleaned after use, and stored in a clean, dry condition.

11. All spilled materials (liquids or powders, or breakages) should be cleaned up in a way that will minimize the possibility of creating further contamination. Again, dry brushing should be avoided and wet and/or vacuum methods employed instead. If there is a risk of microbial contamination, the cleaned area or surface should then be disinfected. Any spillage material that represents a microbiological hazard should be placed in a container, immersed in disinfectant, covered, and removed from the room.

CLEANING OF EQUIPMENT

Between batches, all manufacturing equipment and vessels must be thoroughly cleaned and (as necessary) disinfected or sterilized.

There should be written procedures for doing this, and they must be followed EXACTLY. Each different piece of equipment has its own particular areas where there is a risk, given the right conditions, of microbial growth.

The best modern equipment is usually designed and built to reduce these risks as far as possible. It should:

• Be easy to dismantle and clean;

• Have internal surfaces that are smooth, continuous, with no pits or rough, unpolished welds;

and

• Have no dead-legs, water, or dirt traps.

It may be necessary to strip (or partially strip) equipment down before cleaning it. The written Standard Procedure should always be followed. Often, equipment is mobile, so that it can be removed from the manufacturing room for cleaning in a Wash Bay.

Once equipment has been cleaned and disinfected, or sterilized, steps should be taken to ensure that it cannot become recontaminated. Care must also be taken to ensure (by labeling and/or segregation) that there is no possibility of mix-up between items that have been cleaned and disinfected or sterilized, and those that have not.

7. CONTROL OF CONTAMINATION—WATER AND OTHER MATERIALS

We have already dealt with a number of different aspects of contamination. There is one more we need to consider—that is, the contamination that may be on, or in, the materials we use. Let us first talk briefly about the containers in which we finally pack our products.

CONTAINERS

Things like bottles, ampules, vials, tubes, and syringes must all, of course, be clean, and kept clean—very. It is no use at all manufacturing a very clean, or sterile, bulk product, and then filling or packing it into a dirty bottle, vial, or other container. If a product is not sterilized after it has been filled into its final pack, then the containers will have to be sterilized before they are filled. And, of course, there could be the problem of pyrogens on the surfaces of containers, so again it's a case of ensuring that everything is kept clean, very clean, all along the line.

Cardboard or fiberboard boxes, such as those that might be used for final outer packaging of products or for the supply of materials, should not be allowed in Clean Rooms at all. Not only are they likely to be bearers of microorganisms, they can cause contamination by huge numbers of fibers.

MATERIALS

The actual chemical and other materials used to make the product itself should not contain significant levels of microorganisms or pyrogens. It is usual for manufacturers of Sterile Products to set strict specifications for the microbiological (as well as the chemical) quality of the materials they buy and use. They also carry out laboratory checks on the quality of those materials as they are received from the supplier. It is therefore very important that such materials are not allowed to become contaminated during storage and use.

WATER

Water is by far the biggest volume ingredient used in the manufacture of many Sterile Products. Water is also is widely used
in a variety of washing and rinsing operations. Since water is
so important, and because there are special requirements for
the water used in Sterile Products manufacture (both as an
ingredient and for washing), it is worth spending some time
on WATER alone. Remember, too, that water (moisture) is one
of the three main requirements for microbial growth. That is a
big problem with water—preventing and controlling the
growth of microorganisms that can all too easily happen.

There are a number of different grades of water (in to addition
just plain dirty water!).

For our purposes, we can say that the main grades are:

• Potable Water,

• Purified Water,

and

• Water for Injections.

Quality standard specifications for all these are printed in a
number of official publications.

Potable Water

Potable Water is the ordinary drinking water that emerges from
the mains, through faucets in our homes. Although it is fit to
drink, it is not usually considered suitable for the manufacture
of pharmaceutical products generally, particularly not for
Sterile Products. Most particularly, it is not suitable for the
manufacture of injections. The problem is, ordinary Potable
Water contains quite a wide range of dissolved solids and

gases, which may be harmless when swallowed, but that could be harmful if they were injected. They could also interact with other ingredients in the product. Fine solids are often also found suspended in Potable Water. Also present in most Potable Waters are relatively small amounts of microorganisms. No problem, normally, if drunk straight from the faucet, but unacceptable in Sterile Products. Potable Water is adequate for washing hands in changing rooms, and for some initial washing and rinsing operations. For other uses, we need purer grades of water.

Purified Water

Specifications for Purified Water appear in the *Unites States Pharmacopeia* and in other national and international pharmacopoeias. They all specify chemical purity limits. Purified Water is not necessarily sterile, and is therefore not suitable for the manufacture of injections. It is usually prepared from Potable Water by deionization (a process similar to water-softening), which removes many dissolved substances, but can have the effect of increasing the microbial content. It may also be produced by distillation, or by another process called Reverse Osmosis. Purified Water is not suitable as a constituent of injectable products but, given good control to maintain a low level of microorganisms, it may be used for the initial stages of washing and rinsing the surfaces of equipment and containers that come into contact with the product. For the final rinsing of these surfaces, a higher standard of water is required, which also should be free from pyrogens where the manufacture of injections is involved.

Water for Injections

Standards for Water for Injections also appear in the United States, and other, pharmacopoeias. It is prepared from Potable or Purified Water by a process of distillation. In any event, it is usual to deionize Potable Water before it is distilled. One reason is to prevent the still "scaling-up" like a domestic kettle.

This preliminary deionization removes many of the dissolved substances. Another reason is in line with general philosophy of making Sterile Products—EXTRA SPECIAL CARE at all stages. The higher the quality of the water we feed to a still, the greater the assurance that the still will produce water of the required quality.

Water for Injections is of a very high chemical purity, and is free from pyrogens. When talking about the microbiological quality of Water For Injection, it is necessary to make a distinction between Water For Injections in bulk, and Water For Injections as sold and supplied in ampules or vials for use in making up injections (from powders or freeze-dried material) just immediately before they are injected. In this second case the water MUST be sterile (as well as pyrogen-free). Where Water for Injection is held or supplied in bulk, intended for use in the manufacture of products *that will be sterilized later*, then it need not be sterile. It is, however, very important that its level of microorganisms is kept very low.

Once again, it is all about that EXTRA CARE, all along the line. The lower the level of organisms in the product or material to be sterilized, the greater the assurance of the success of the sterilization process.

The process of distillation is, in essence, a very simple one. The water is heated to its boiling point, the resultant water vapor, or steam, is condensed, and the condensate (or distillate) is collected.

In practice, things get more complicated. One important consideration is to design the still so as to prevent the carryover ("entrainment" is the word often used) of fine droplets of water that may contain dissolved solids, particles, and pyrogens, and thus defeat the whole object. The main reason for the different variations of still design are to prevent this from happening, and also to make them more efficient (in terms of output) and cost-effective. (Distillation is a costly business, requiring a high energy input.)

Holding and Distribution of Water

It is no use producing high quality Water for Injections, and then allowing it to become recontaminated. Remember, microorganisms LOVE water—a few organisms in water today will become many millions tomorrow, if the conditions are favorable for them. There are a number of ways of using, holding, or distributing water once it has been distilled.

These include:

1. Using the water immediately and directly upon collection from the still. This eliminates the need for any storage or distribution system, but is really only applicable to small-scale production.

2. Collecting the water in a clean vessel that is then sealed and sterilized in an autoclave (see the next section on Sterilization). This means the water can be stored for a considerable period, but is again only appropriate to very small-scale production.

3. Collecting the water, piped direct from the still, in a sealed holding tank designed and insulated so as to keep the water at a temperature above 80°C. Water is then taken, or pumped, from the tank as required.

4. The best system, and the one commonly used in large-scale Sterile Manufacture, is to connect this type of holding tank to a ring-main piping system in which the water is continuously circulated, from and back to the holding tank at a temperature above 80°C. (Although 80°C will not necessarily kill all species of microorganisms, it will kill many of them, and discourage the growth and reproduction of the others.)

Other Types of Water

In addition to Potable Water, Purified Water, and Water For Injection, you may come across other types of water. For example, there is water used for cooling equipment. It is not usual to specify standards for such water, provided it does not come into contact with product, or with surfaces that will, in turn, contact the product. It is important to note that water of this nonspecified quality is NOT suitable for use as water for cooling product following sterilization in an autoclave.

Another type is Boiler Feed Water. Again, if such water does not come into contact, directly or indirectly, with the product or its environment, then its chemical and microbiological quality is not too important. But "ordinary" Boiler Feed Water, which often contains chemical substances that have been deliberately added to it, is NOT suitable for use to make steam for the sterilization of products, containers, or processing equipment.

For steam that will be in contact with products or in contact with surfaces that products will in turn contact, we need Clean Steam. Clean Steam is produced in specially designed Clean Steam Generators, from Purified or Distilled Water. The essential feature of Clean Steam is that when it condenses, it should form Water for Injections quality water.

The quality of Water (and of any steam made from it) that is required depends on its use and on the nature of the things or surfaces with which it will come into contact. The Golden Rule about water is:

It is vital always to use the right defined-quality water as specified for the purpose.

8. STERILIZATION

We have so far talked about a number of different ways of controlling contamination. We now come to the ultimate in microbial contamination control—STERILIZATION—that is, the complete destruction or removal of living things. Make no mistake about it. We are not talking half measures. Sterilization means killing or removing all forms of life. The lot. Period.

There are a number of different methods of sterilization, and we use one or other of them to sterilize products, and also the containers, vessels, equipment, and pipes with which they may be in contact.

Broadly speaking, there are two different, basic approaches to making a Sterile Product:

1. Filling and sealing the product into its final container and then sterilizing it. This is called "TERMINAL STERILIZATION."

2. Sterilizing a product at some earlier stage, before it is filled or packed, and then carrying out further processing and filling into sterile containers, using ASEPTIC techniques and taking ASEPTIC precautions—that is, using special techniques to avoid recontamination.

If possible, it is best to use a Terminal Sterilization process, simply because if the product is sterilized when securely sealed in its container, then it will remain sterile until the container is opened, broken, or punctured in some way. When working with an unsealed Sterile Product, there is always a risk of recontamination. That risk, however, can be greatly reduced if the proper care is taken. Nevertheless, most experts and regulatory authorities agree that, where it is possible, products should be terminally sterilized. (Sometimes this is not possible, for example, when a product is not able to withstand a terminal heat sterilization process.)

Always, once something has been sterilized, very great care must be taken to ensure that it does not become recontaminated, or mixed up with nonsterile items.

METHODS OF STERILIZATION

First, one important general **Golden Rule:**

Whatever type of sterilization process is used, the existing procedures MUST be followed precisely, every time. There is no room for minor variations, or for playing it by ear, or doing it by the seat of your pants.

The main methods of Sterilization are as follows:

- **Heat, either**
  - **Moist (that is, Steam)**
  - or
  - **Dry.**

- **Radiation (for example, Gamma Rays or Electron Beams).**

- **Gas (for example, Ethylene Oxide).**

- **Filtration.**

There are other methods, but these are the ones most often used. The objective is the same in all cases—to get rid of microorganisms, but the various methods used are all very different from each other. For example, in at least one important respect, filtration is different from all the other methods. Sterilization by heat, radiation, or gas kills microorganisms. Filtration removes them.

Heat Sterilization

Sterilization by heat is usually the best method. The main reason for choosing *not* to use a heat sterilization process would be when the product or material cannot stand the heat required and would, therefore, break down or deteriorate.

Of the two possible forms of heat sterilization, moist heat (that is Steam) is usually better, and more effective at lower temperatures. The reasons for this are the better contact (and thus heat transfer) that the steam provides, and the fact that steam has a greater content of heat energy than, say, hot air at the same temperature.

Steam Sterilization

Steam sterilization is used to sterilize aqueous (watery) solutions in sealed containers, such as bottles, vials, or ampules. It is also used to sterilize water-wettable articles, such as containers, instruments, some medical devices, and also machine and equipment parts.

When sterilizing things like containers, instruments, or machine parts, it is essential that precautions are taken to prevent recontamination after the sterilization process has been completed. This may be done, for example, by wrapping the item to be sterilized in bags or sheets of special material that allows the removal of air and the penetration of steam, but that form a barrier against entry of microorganisms after the sterilization. Often, two layers of the material are used (the "double wrapping" technique). This enables successive removal of the two layers, while, for example, the sterilized item is passed through a hatchway into a Clean Room, with the inner wrapping only removed when the sterilized item is under some form of protection against recontamination (such as a Laminar Air Flow cabinet).

Steam Sterilization is not a suitable method for the sterilization of sealed containers of oily solutions or suspensions. The reason is that the special effectiveness of Steam Sterilization is due to the moist, not dry, heat. Oily material in a sealed container may reach the temperature of the steam sterilizing chamber, but the heat will only be dry heat and that (at the temperatures usually used for steam sterilization) will not be sufficient.

It is important to know that boiling water (or steam) at normal atmospheric pressure (that is, water or steam at 100°C) will not kill all organisms. It will kill many, even most, of them. But some microorganisms are amazingly tough, particularly those that can form spores. Some of these spore-formers are very dangerous, and can survive boiling in water for long periods. Therefore, while in certain cases it may be considered safe to drink slightly contaminated water after boiling, higher temperatures are needed to ensure true sterilization. To achieve these higher steam temperatures, it is necessary to operate under pressure, in equipment that is similar in principle to a pressure cooker, that is, in autoclaves.

One of the most commonly used combinations of temperature and time is 121°C for 15 minutes. Other combinations of temperature and time may be used, provided that they have been shown to achieve the desired result. For example:

Temperature (°C)	Time (minutes)
115–118	30
121–124	15
126–129	10
134–138	3

Important points to note are:

- As the temperature increases, the time required reduces significantly.

- The temperate must be achieved throughout the load for the time required. For example, if a temperature of 121°C for 15 minutes is used, then this temperature must be achieved at the coldest part of the coldest item in the coldest section of the load for at least 15 minutes. It is

NOT sufficient that at some point, or points, this temperature is achieved for the specified time.

- The pressure is only used to achieve the required temperature, and contributes nothing to the sterilization process. It is the temperature that is the important thing. It must be used to control and monitor the process.

Dry Heat

This is the method used in hot air ovens or sterilizing tunnels.

Because dry heat is less effective in sterilization than steam, higher temperatures and longer exposure times are required. Again, it is vital that all parts of all items being sterilized reach at least the required temperature for at least the required time.

Time/temperature combinations for DRY HEAT sterilization that are generally accepted as effective are:

Temperature (°C)	Time (minutes)
180	30
170	60
160	120

Radiation Sterilization

Another method of killing microorganisms is by exposure to some form of radiation.

Sterilization by such irradiation methods can be very effective, especially since it can be used to sterilize products and materials that are already packaged, provided the radiation can penetrate the package. In these circumstances, it is a means of terminal sterilization without the use of heat. A problem is that radiation can cause serious deterioration of a number of products, materials, compounds, and containers. Also, very expensive and complex plants and equipment are required. Most Sterile Products manufacturers who have products or materials sterilized by radiation send them out to a limited number of specialist organizations that do this work under contract.

Gas Sterilization

Many chemical substances are toxic to microorganisms, but only a very limited number of them have any use as sterilizing agents (as distinct from the variety of chemical substances that can be effectively used as disinfectants).

While other substances have been proposed and tried, in practice, the substance that has been most widely used as a sterilant is the gas Ethylene Oxide.

Ethylene Oxide can only be used to sterilize surfaces. That is, unlike heat or radiation, it cannot penetrate through the walls of many containers to the product inside. (It is therefore not possible, for example, to sterilize sealed vials or ampules of product by Ethylene Oxide, although it will penetrate certain plastic films and bags.)

Among the disadvantages of Ethylene Oxide is that it is highly flammable—explosive even (it is usually used diluted with an inert gas)—and is highly toxic to people. For these and other reasons, its use is declining.

Filtration Sterilization

While, as we have said, all the different sterilization processes are different from each other, Filtration is "more different" from all the rest. That is because it:

- Removes organisms rather than killing them

and

- Is only applicable to fluids (liquids and gases).

It also cannot be used as a terminal sterilization process. Any sterile-filtered bulk product that is not going to be subjected to a further terminal sterilization must be filled and sealed into final containers observing special ("ASEPTIC") precautions to prevent recontamination. Thus, a further element of risk is involved. That is why it is generally considered that, where it is possible to terminally heat-sterilize products (particularly injections), this should be done, with filtration sterilization restricted to use where the product, or its container, cannot withstand heating. However, more modern and automated techniques such as "Barrier" or "Blow/Fill/Seal" technology are being increasingly refined and used to significantly reduce the risks of recontamination following sterilization by Filtration.

In essence, sterilization by filtration is a simple process. A liquid is forced, under moderate pressure, through a filter that is in the form of a membrane or cartridge, the filter itself and the assembly in which it is mounted having been sterilized previously. As the liquid passes through it, the filter holds back and retains any microorganisms or other fine particles.

Various types, sizes, grades and pore-sizes of filter are available from a number of specialist manufacturers. Given the right filter for the job, properly assembled, fitted, and sterilized, and with confirmation that the filter is not damaged before use (or has not become damaged during use), it is possible to attain a very high level of assurance that the liquid is sterile as it emerges through the filter. Tests must be carried out to confirm that the filter is not damaged or punctured and that it was properly fitted in its holder. This is done to ensure that all the liquid is filtered—that some has not passed through a hole or split in the filter, or has not been able to "creep" around it. These tests are called "Filter Integrity Tests."

But, as we have said, the main problem is to ensure that the liquid does not become recontaminated after the filtration. That is not easy, particularly where people are involved. That is why sterilization by filtration, although it seems a simple business, is the method that demands the utmost care and attention.

Whatever method of sterilization is used, it is VITAL to get it right, every time. That is, it really is a matter of life and death to be certain that what we are sterilizing does in fact end up, and stay, sterile. And that means that there are no living organisms in or on it. People can be, and have been, killed because products that were supposed to be sterile were not.

With these thoughts in mind, we can set out some:

RULES ABOUT STERILIZATION

1. **Sterilization means the elimination (by killing or removal) of ALL living organisms, and great care and attention is needed to ensure that this is achieved.**

2. **Different methods of sterilization are used for different purposes. The method that is specified in the manufacturing instructions is the one that must be used, and only that one.**

3. **The official written procedure MUST be followed, exactly, every time.**

4. **If anything unusual happens, or if there are any deviations from the official written procedure, then it all must be recorded and reported, so that a decision can be made on whether or not the sterilization was successful. (REMEMBER—we just cannot rely on the Sterility Test alone.)**

5. When a liquid is sterilized by filtration, then it is necessary to confirm the integrity of the filter assembly. Very great care is also necessary to ensure that the liquid does not become recontaminated.

6. It is VITAL to ensure that things (products, materials, equipment) that have been sterilized cannot become mixed up with things that have not. They should be kept well segregated from one another, and be marked or labeled in some way to indicate whether they are sterile or not.

9. CONCLUSION

This booklet has been about the manufacture of Sterile Products. In particular, it has been about the very special care that is necessary at all stages in their manufacture.

All products for medical use need to be made in accordance with the basic principles of Good Manufacturing Practice (GMP). When such products are intended to be injected, inserted, or implanted into blood vessels or other tissues, or into body cavities, or to be used in eyes or on wounds, then they must be sterile. That means that, in addition to all the usual GMP precautions, there is a whole range of additional things that require extra care and attention. This booklet was written to help you understand what these things are. Its most important message is that so much depends on the people who make these products. In a very real sense, other people's lives are in your hands.

APPENDIX A—CLEAN ROOMS

Much of the manufacture and filling of Sterile Products, and certainly all those stages where there is any possibility that the product or its container could become contaminated, is carried out in Clean Rooms, or at least within confined areas that have a defined and controlled level of microbial (viable) and particulate contamination.

Remember that a CLEAN ROOM in this special sense is not just a room that is clean. It is a room that is classifiable into one or other of several Classes or Grades of "clean-ness."

The concept and design of Clean Rooms was first developed in 1964 for the microelectronic and aerospace industries. In these, it is important to protect microelectronic components against even the finest particles. Living contaminants, as such, are of no special significance to microcircuits, only in so far as bacteria are themselves particles.

Because of these origins, in industries where sterility as such is not the aim, the classification of the various Classes of Clean Room is based on the number and size of the particles permitted in the air in the room. (The published Clean Room standards also have specifications for humidity, temperature, lighting, and air pressure.) It was only later that the Pharmaceutical Industry took over the idea, and then added to it, in some cases, certain permissible levels of microbial (viable) contamination.

So, it is first necessary to understand the numerical basis of the classification of Clean Rooms.

The unit used to measure fine particles is called a "MICROMETER," or "MICRON." In fact, the term most commonly used is "micron." A micron (or micrometer) is 1/1000th (0.001) of a millimeter, or one millionth of a meter. (For those who prefer to think in inches, it is about 39 millionths of an inch). An idea of the size of a micron can be gained from Figure Y on the next page:

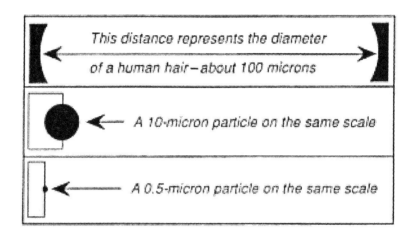

Figure Y The size of a micron, as compared to a human hair.

The first widely accepted official published standard for Clean Rooms was the United States's "Federal Standard 209: Clean Room and Work Station Requirements, Controlled Environment." This has gone through a number of revisions over the years since the 1960s (the latest is Federal Standard 209E, first published in 1992), but the basic ideas behind the classification remain the same. The standard is largely based on permitted numbers, per CUBIC FOOT of air in a room, of particles of a size 0.5 micron and larger.

For our purposes, we need to think only of three main Classes of Clean Room—Class 100, Class 10,000, and Class 100,000, and it works like this:

Federal Standard 209 Clean Room Standards
*Maximum Permitted Number of Particles
per Cubic Foot of Air in Room:*

	0.5 micron & larger	5.0 micron & larger
Class 100	100	0
Class 10,000	10,000	65
Class 100,000	100,000	700

The latest revision of the Standard (that is, 209E) also provides equivalent figures for the permitted number of particles per cubic *meter* of air.

This Standard defines a number of other aspects of Clean Rooms, such as temperature, humidity, air pressure, operator clothing, and the instruments and devices used to measure and count nonviable particles in the air. So, although Clean Rooms are classified on the basis of the number of particles permitted per cubic foot (or per cubic meter) of the air in the room, there are a number of other important items that require attention. For example, the US Current Good Manufacturing Practice Regulations ("the **cGMPs**") state, in **Subpart C—Buildings and Facilities:**

Sec. 211.42 Design and construction features

. . .

(c) . . .

(10) Aseptic processing, which includes as appropriate:

(i) Floors, walls and ceilings of smooth, hard surfaces that are easily cleanable

(ii) Temperature and humidity controls

(iii) An air supply filtered through high-efficiency particulate air filters . . .

(iv) A system for monitoring environmental conditions

(v) A system for cleaning and disinfecting the room and equipment . . .

(vi) A system for maintaining any equipment used to control the aseptic conditions.

There is also the area that is perhaps the most important aspect of Clean Rooms used for sterile products manufacture. That is the reduction and control of microbial (viable) contamination. You remember that Clean Rooms were originally developed for use in the microelectronics and aerospace industries, where specifically viable contamination is no big issue. In the manufacture of sterile products, it is a very big issue indeed—even more significant than nonviable particles. Although it is important to keep particles out of, or off of, our sterile products, it is even more important that we prevent them from being contaminated with microorganisms. If we don't, they won't be sterile! Internationally, there has been much discussion on acceptable standards for permitted levels of viable in Clean Rooms. That discussion continues. The following table is given as an illustration of the sort of standards for viable contamination adopted by many manufacturers of sterile products, expressed as allowable numbers per cubic meter of air:

Clean Room Class	Maximum permitted number of microorganisms per cubic meter of air
Cl. 100	less than 1
Cl. 10,000	not more than 5
Cl. 100,000	not more than 100

There are a number of techniques that are used to monitor the number of microorganisms (viables) in a Clean Room. There are a number of mechanical devices that sample the air and enable the viables to be counted. A simple and widely used method is to expose petri dishes of a nutrient gel ("settle plates") for a specified time, and then incubate them. The number of microbial colonies that then form can be counted to give an indication of the number of microorganisms that have been deposited from the air in the time specified. Surfaces in the room can be monitored by the use of bacterial swabs or contact plates.

T - #1038 - 101024 - C0 - 216/138/4 - PB - 9781574911343 - Gloss Lamination